I0413408

Flat Belly Diet
For Women:

How to Lose Belly
Fat Fast and Easy

By

Barbara Moore

ISBN-13: 978-1495493942

Table of Contents

Flat Belly Diet For Women: How to Lose Belly Fat Fast and
Easy

By Barbara Moore

First Published, 2013

Printed in the United States of America

Introduction

On an average day in America at least 50% of women over the age of 18 are on a diet. In fact, 80% of women say they are dissatisfied with their bodies and want to lose weight. It should be easy given the theory that burning more calories than you take in results in weight loss but unfortunately, women's bodies work against them with stubborn determination.

This book Flat Belly Diet For Women: How to Lose Belly Fat Fast and Easy is here to help you to get a flat belly and fit body.

Chapter 1. Why it's Hard for Women to Lose Belly Fat

Women have a unique problem when it comes to belly fat because of the way the female body is engineered—it hoards fat, not just because of the threat of famine but because it may be called upon to nourish another human being for about 30-35 years a woman's life. Unfortunately, the modern woman's body is about five thousand years behind social progress; it is always prepared for starvation and no amount of plenty will convince it that life has become relatively free of deprivation. That's why women can follow the same advice men get for a flat belly and still not achieve their goals.

Not only is the female body different metabolically but fat looks different on women than it does on men. A man can carry ten, fifteen, or even twenty pounds of extra fat and still look attractive because of their size and the way they are built. Women, with their smaller frames and curves, show every extra pound that their bodies so eagerly accumulate and that weight usually settles into the hips and belly. Clothing clings in all the wrong places, even the looser styles that become popular every few years. Ironically, hip and belly fat are the hardest to get rid of and many women eventually resign themselves to larger sizes or disguising styles.

It doesn't have to be that way if you understand how your body works, what it needs to stay in shape, and how you can persuade it to burn belly fat to get the slim, healthy body every woman wants.

Chapter 2. Losing Belly Fat Means Eating Differently

When you go on a diet to lose belly fat or generally trim your body you are dooming yourself to failure. This may sound illogical but it is true, especially if you are female. Depriving the body of the fuel it is used to is like telling a person they won't have water for three days—they pour and store all the water they can get their hands on. Your body does the same thing with the fat already in the body and any fuel coming in, storing and hoarding it until the "famine" is over. And the best place, according to genetic wisdom, to keep that precious fat is in the belly, hips, and thighs. Any energy expended for the everyday needs of living is automatically withdrawn from breasts, arms, and healthy muscle tissue; the body does this in order to preserve enough fat to make it through until the calories start increase enough that the body believes things are back to normal.

This is the reason why you might lose a few pounds the first week of a diet then reach a plateau or stop losing altogether. The key to losing fat in general and getting that flat belly you want is to work with your body instead of against it. This means adopting a different style of eating rather than drastically cutting calories.

Chapter 3. Adopting a Saner Eating Style

Rather than encourage your body to store fat by cutting way down on calories you can start your flat belly program by cutting out a hundred calories a day. This could be giving up your morning toast, forgoing the crackers with your cheese, or eating half a regular serving of pasta for dinner. The calories you're giving up are simple carbohydrates, something your body has little use for but loves for their fat building qualities. The calories you're saving are not enough to set off alarms and cause your body to shift into fat-hoarding mode but it is enough to re-educate it to accept fewer simple carbs and calories.

After a week or so of getting your body used to fewer calories it's time to change the foods you are eating. Did you ever wonder why it was rare to see an obese person just fifty years ago? The average person didn't work out (in fact, gyms were rare in the mid-60's) or have a particularly active lifestyle but they ate quite differently than we do today. Going to the store and filling your cart with "healthy" frozen meals was a concept for science fiction movies. There were very few frozen vegetables and you ordered meat from the butcher counter, freshly cut or ground, using it that very day because there were no preservatives to keep it fresh in the refrigerator for days.

The best thing you can do to get that flat belly and svelte thighs you want is to return to the simpler eating style that your body was built for. Our bodies were not made to ingest chemicals, preservatives, dyes, pesticides and growth hormones that are found in meats and, to a lesser extent, vegetables and fruits.

Chapter 4. Eating For a Flat Belly

So, what can you eat? And won't it take time that you don't have? Not necessarily—in fact, you may even save some time! You'll certainly be eating a healthier diet and adding years to your life!

If you haven't already joined the organic bandwagon, now is a good time to do so. Sure, organic meats and produce cost more— sometimes a lot more!—but the health benefits outweigh the monetary outlay. Most people notice a change in their bodies and their energy levels as they stop ingesting all the additives in meats, produce and frozen foods. Plus, organic meat comes from animals that are allowed to move around naturally instead of being inhumanely caged in areas so small that they cannot move. Most people say that they can taste the difference, too. As your body adjusts to the more natural food your metabolism will also adjust. It will be able to devote more energy to everyday functions rather than fighting small inflammations caused by the unnatural foreign elements in today's common foods.

Balance is Everything

It is important to have a healthy, balanced diet if you want to get that flat belly and slim body. Limiting yourself to just a few foods that you can make quickly and conveniently will put you in a rut, one that will lull your body into a routine that guarantees it won't make efficient use of the calories you give it. It won't make a big dent in your schedule, either, but that will be addressed later.

One simple way to make sure you're giving your body the nourishment it needs without extra calories it doesn't is to divide your plate into fractions. One fourth should be lean protein such as baked, broiled, or steamed fish, crustaceans like crab, beef, pork, poultry and the like. Another fourth should be filled with complex carbs such as whole grain breads, legumes, or other unrefined carbs. Half your plate should consist of leafy greens and vegetables, the more colorful the better.

Zucchini, squash, green beans, eggplant, carrots and other bright plants will provide fiber, vitamins, and minerals your body needs and very few calories. If you like dessert for dinner you can eat a serving of fruit and occasionally a small piece of cake or serving of ice cream.

Portion it Correctly

One of the reasons why diets fail is because people feel deprived. While eating organic foods and a balanced, varied menu is a great way to get a flat belly, you're going to have cravings for your favorite treats—there's no way out of that, no matter what kind of supplements you take or how much will power you have! The key is to read the label, find out how much a portion is—and measure it! Most people spoon out what they think is a ½ cup serving of ice cream but they would find, if they measured what they dished out, that it is close to or exceeds that portion by half or more!

There is nothing wrong with indulging yourself occasionally. It won't sabotage your diet and in not depriving yourself you'll head off any overwhelming cravings you may develop and avoid binge eating.

You should measure all your food, even if you use the divided plate method. It's not that inconvenient and insures that you're accurately counting your calories, fat, carbs, and protein units.

Sample Menus for a Flat Belly

Breakfast is the meal that tells your body it's okay to start burning calories again so be sure you don't skip this important meal. A good breakfast should include complex carbs such as whole grain cereal or oatmeal. You could have a breakfast muffin from a batch you made on the weekend with oat bran, an egg, berries or other fruit, nuts, and cinnamon. Breakfast should also include yogurt, cottage cheese, milk, or another dairy product and fruit or fruit juice. Having an egg a few times a week is actually good for you no matter what the cholesterol alarmists claim; eggs are a great source of protein and vitamins that few other foods can mimic.

For lunch you can have a salad or use the greens in a pita or a sandwich made with lean meat. Fat free mayonnaise may not sound good but it makes a delicious chicken/ham/tuna salad with greatly reduced calories and all the taste. Lunch is a good time to have a serving of dairy whether you enjoy a cube of cheese or have a slice on a sandwich. Just be sure to avoid white bread. If you have a microwave at your job, or if you work at home, you can even heat up last night's leftover entrée and add a leafy green salad.

Most people look at dinner as their reward for a hard days' work, and why not? Dinner should be special, a prelude to a relaxing evening walk or bike ride followed by winding down for the night. This should not be a heavy meal (you'll sleep better!) but cover all the food groups in small portions. Crab legs, broiled chicken, or a small steak broiled with onions and mushrooms will provide protein. You can serve it with eggplant or butternut squash, a couple of small red potatoes or brown rice, green beans with almonds, and/or a salad of leafy greens.

One of the keys to a successful diet and flat belly is variety!

Chapter 5. Cooking For a Flat Belly

Just because you give up frozen and processed foods doesn't mean you have to give up convenience and spend all of your time cooking. Nearly everyone can find an hour or two during a day off to prepare their week's food then store or freeze it for later use.

You can start with the breakfast muffins mentioned earlier. While they are baking you can broil some poultry, divide it into individual portions and refrigerate or freeze them. Add them to brown rice, pasta, or other dishes later in the week. As for the pasta, you can make it ahead of time and *lightly* coat it with olive oil before refrigerating or freezing it. You'll find that it the taste and texture is just as pleasing when you microwave it from the freezer as when you cook it up fresh.

After you cook and store your meat and make some breakfast muffins to put in the fridge or to freeze, you can divide salad into daily portions. If you wrap salad in tin foil or Glad brand Press 'n Seal it will stay fresh and crisp for at least ten days. You can take a portion out for dinner or pack it in your lunch tote.

Having spent an hour or so cooking and storing your week's food, all you have to do each day is microwave most things while you cook your fresh vegetables.

Cool Ginger Tea

Ginger has a powerful digestive benefits plus will also improve heath of the immune system. This is a recipe that is made from ginger tea bags and other ingredients that are known to help women acquire the hourglass figure they are looking for.

You need about 3 ginger tea bags, a cup of fresh mint coarsely chopped, a tablespoon of fresh lemon juice, about 2 cups of water and ice. Use a large 24-ounce pitcher to make your fresh ginger tea. Steep the bags of tea and mint for about 10 minutes and then strain to remove the mint leaves and the tea bags. Afterwards add the tablespoon of lemon juice and stir. Place this in the refrigerator until chilled. Serve with ice. You can sip a glass of ginger tea as often as you wish in a day until you have consumed the entire contents of the pitcher. If you would like to share your drink, double the ingredients to make another pitcher-full of cool ginger tea drink.

Breakfast Fruit and Nut Oatmeal Treat

Breakfast is the most important meal of the day and what better way to start a flat belly diet recipe. Three important foods that promote a flat belly are in this breakfast treat: berries, nuts and oats. You need 2/3 cup of old-fashioned oatmeal, ¾ frozen strawberries and a tablespoon of pecan nuts.

Simply cook oatmeal in water to your desired consistency. Warm the berries in a microwave or take it out of the deep freeze before you cook your oatmeal. When the oatmeal is done, top it with strawberries and a tablespoon of pecan nuts. Eating these flat belly foods will help keep you feeling fuller for a longer period of time and prevent you from snacking before lunch time.

Salmon on Whole Wheat Bread

Salmon is a perfect source of protein; this recipe is a salmon sandwich on whole wheat which is a great lunchtime favorite to flatten your belly fast. You need 2 pieces of whole wheat bread seasoned with sesame seeds, 2 tablespoons of black olive tapenade, a can (3oz) Alaskan salmon, romaine lettuce leaves and diced plum tomato.

Spread the tapenade over 2 pieces of whole wheat bread and then place the salmon pieces on top. Add the diced plum tomatoes and a couple of romaine lettuce leaves. Make and share your sandwich with a friend by simply doubling the recipe ingredients.

Delicious Chicken Pasta and Cheese

This is a recipe that you may prepare for dinner or for a special occasion. You need 1/3 cup whole wheat pasta cooked according to package instructions, a tablespoon of pesto sauce, about 3 ounces of cooked and fillet chicken breast, ½ cup of grape tomatoes, a tablespoon of grated cheese and ½ cup of shredded carrots.

Simply toss the ingredients together and place a tablespoon of pesto sauce all over the dish. You may add more tomatoes and more cheese over the dish if you want or double maybe triple the ingredients if you want to share this flat belly dish with your friends.

Meatball Cheese Melt

This recipe may be for lunch or for dinner but would be great when partnered with whole wheat pasta. You need a piece of multigrain pita bread, veggie meatballs 2 pieces, a tablespoon of Italian cheeses blend shredded, extra virgin olive oil and marinara sauce.

Prepare the pita bread on a plate, place the meatballs on top of the bread and drizzle with olive oil and about ½ tablespoon of marinara sauce. Top this meaty recipe with 4 cheeses blend and serve hot. If you wish to serve it with whole wheat pasta, cook about 1/3 cup according to package instructions. Drizzle the pasta with extra virgin olive oil and marinara sauce and add the two meatballs on top of the pasta. Top everything with cheese and serve hot.

Tuna Melt on Whole Grain Bread

Just like salmon, tuna is a rich source of protein which helps build muscles and tissues. This recipe is a lunch time favorite that you will also love to serve for dinner. You need a slice of whole grain bread, a small can of light tuna in water, a tablespoon of sunflower seeds and shredded parmesan cheese.

Green Mexicali Salad

Green veggies will help keep you full for a long period of time plus adds fiber to your diet that cleans the gastrointestinal system. This ingredients call for 2 cups of baby greens mixed, ½ cup beans, green chilies, ¾ cups sweet corn kernels, ¼ cup red onion sliced, ¼ cup of salsa and about ¼ cup sliced avocado.

Combine all the ingredients together in a large bowl and toss. Drizzle with salsa and then toss once more. Double all the ingredients if you want to make salad for two. Other ingredients that can make this salad greener are green sprouts, string green beans and so many more. You may also change the salsa salad dressing into extra virgin olive oil.

Veggie Burger in Pita Bread

Veggie burger is a burger made from meat substitute. This recipe calls for a medium to large multi-grain pita bread, a veggie burger, ½ cup baby spinach, 2 tablespoons of scallions and 4 cups of sliced avocados. Chop the veggie burger into smaller pieces and then combine all the ingredients in a bowl. Remove the inner portion of pita bread and then stuff it with the mixture. Heat this in a microwave oven. Serve the stuffed pita bread warm along with a green salad for lunch or dinner.

Salmon steak dinner

This is a protein boost for dinner; this dish tastes great and is very nutritious too. You need a piece of wild Alaskan salmon steak seasoned with freshly ground pepper and salt. As a side dish, cook green beans in a microwave oven. Serve the salmon steak with pepper and sliced almonds. You may also toss green Mexicali salad as an appetizer to compliment this delicious dish.

Cheese on Toast

This is a crunchy cheese sandwich that you can eat for breakfast or for snacks. You need sesame-sprouted whole grain bread, 1/8 cup of ricotta cheese and 2 tablespoons of chopped walnuts. Place ricotta cheese on bread and chopped walnuts on whole grain bread. Place this in an oven toaster to toast the bread and melt the cheese.

Banana and Strawberry Oatmeal

Do you want your oatmeal to be creamier and sweeter? This is a recipe that calls for, ½ cup of old-fashioned oatmeal, ripe bananas, ¼ cup of frozen strawberries, a tablespoon of semisweet chocolate chips and 2 tablespoons of almonds. Cook oatmeal in water until you attained the right consistency; slice the banana into small pieces and cut semisweet chocolate chips. Blend all the ingredients into warm oatmeal and then serve. You may want to make your oatmeal chocolatier by adding more chocolate chips. Double or triple the recipe if you want to cook for your family.

Pita on Eggs

Eggs are handy protein sources that can be made into anything and included in different recipes. Pita on eggs calls for ½ multigrain pita bread, 2 eggs, ½ cup baby spinach, ¼ salsa and ¼ cup avocado. Slice ingredients into very small pieces and fill the pita bread with the mixture. Toast the filled pita bread using a microwave or oven toaster to make the bread crispier.

Pepperoni Pizza

Use multigrain pita bread as pizza crust. Brush the bread with extra virgin olive oil and a dash of marinara sauce. You will also need a cup of veggie pepperoni and Italian four-cheese blend. Place these ingredients over the pita bread with olive oil and marinara sauce and if you want this pizza to be cheesier you may add more cheese. This pepperoni pizza will make a hearty dinner for two. Double the ingredients if you want to make more pizzas for a family of four.

Fruity Fruit Salad

Use fruits in season for this amazing dessert selection. Chop cups of melons, pineapples, strawberries, blueberries and watermelons. Mix these fruits together and don't forget to use low fat cream as a dressing. You must chill this salad in the fridge for about an hour before serving them to your guests or family. You may also place heaping full of fruit mixture in plastic cups and top these cups with frothy and sweet low fat cream. Freeze these fruity cups so you will have a fruity and traditional dessert. Fruits are low in calorie so you can eat fruits as much as you want. You may serve fruits for dessert or you may freeze this for a snack. Fruits will also make you feel fuller so the results are you do not need to eat snacks or in between meals anymore. Fruits will are also very nutritious, these are rich in vitamins like vitamin C, A and D and minerals that are needed by the body for optimum health and development of tissues and cells.

Chapter 7. Dealing with Cravings

Cravings are what sabotages most diets. The problem is that by the time you crave something it becomes an irresistible obsession and you tend to binge. One way to fight cravings is to take a multivitamin each day to make sure you're getting what your body needs. A person usually craves something because their body is lacking a key element in that food. If you crave chocolate, your body may be telling you that it's low on magnesium while if you have a yen for a thick, juicy steak your body may be low on iron.

On the other hand, especially if you're nearing your 40's, you may have a hormonal imbalance that makes you crave sweets or carbohydrates. Now is a good time to have your hormones checked and make a visit to your gynecologist to ensure everything is in balance.

Chapter 8. Exercising to Get That Flat Belly

Crunches and sit-ups are not going to give you that flat belly you want. You'll have strong core muscles to support your spine but such exercise won't do much to make your belly fat disappear. So forget about ordering the latest contraption on the shopping channel with six easy payments of $59.99 because you can exercise more efficiently—and have more fun doing it while you melt off that belly fat.

The fact is, you can't spot-reduce fat. You can't exercise one part of your body and lose inches and shrink fat cells in one place and not another. Our bodies are built to use fat for energy and every body will use the fat not essential for survival first. That means the fat cells in your breasts, arms and legs will shrink before the ones in your belly shrink. But you don't have to look like a stick figure with a large middle if you exercise *smart*.

They way your body uses fat is an infallible argument for weight training. Muscle requires more energy to maintain than do fat cells so the more muscle you build, the faster the fat will be used all over your body including your belly. You won't look masculine or disproportionate and you don't have to join a fitness club unless you really want to because you don't need machines.

Push-ups and wall presses (pushing your weight off the nearest wall) are great for developing toned, healthy arms and they also work your core muscles. Squats, leg lifts, and lunges are wonderful for building and toning muscles in your buttocks, thighs, and calves. You don't need special equipment because you're using your own body weight to work against. A hula hoop is a great, fun way to trim your waist and burn fat all over and a good old-fashioned jump rope is good cardiovascular exercise that will also help maintain your balance skills.

Biking and swimming are excellent workouts that are good for your heart, too, but there's not much that beats walking. In fact, people who walk every day generally are more fit and lose more weight in shorter amounts of time than those that work out exclusively in the gym. Walking works your body all over and has several advantages; it can be solitary or social, the scenery is always changing, you get invigorating fresh air and you get to enjoy the sun's warmth.

You should also know that exposure to sunlight is the only way your body can make vitamin D, a very important vitamin that keeps your heart and bones strong and healthy. Take some sun block if you like and use it after fifteen or twenty minutes. Limit your exposure to ten or fifteen minutes if you're very light complexioned. Any time you're out in the sun and fresh air you'll be giving your body important nutrients as well as exercise.

Chapter 9. Make Realistic Goals

You'll want to keep your goals simple and small so that you don't get discouraged. It took awhile to accumulate that fat and it will take awhile to make it disappear. Setting a goal of ten pounds in your first month will only discourage you and sabotage your new lifestyle; losing a pound a week is realistic and achievable.

Conclusion

Now that you know how to get a flat belly and the trim, healthy body you deserve there's no time like the present to start!

Thank You Page

I want to personally thank you for reading my book. I hope you found information in this book useful and I would be very grateful if you could leave your honest review about this book. I certainly want to thank you in advance for doing this.